Mayara Rodrigues
Manoel Garcia Neto

Minimising broiler mortality

Mayara Rodrigues
Manoel Garcia Neto

Minimising broiler mortality

Electrolyte balance and early heat conditioning

ScienciaScripts

Imprint

Cover image: www.ingimage.com

This book is a translation from the original published under ISBN 978-3-330-76088-2.

Publisher:
Sciencia Scripts
is a trademark of
Dodo Books Indian Ocean Ltd. and OmniScriptum S.R.L publishing group

120 High Road, East Finchley, London, N2 9ED, United Kingdom
Str. Armeneasca 28/1, office 1, Chisinau MD-2012, Republic of Moldova, Europe
Printed at: see last page
ISBN: 978-620-8-34309-5

SUMMARY

ABSTRACT - In countries with a tropical climate, heat is one of the main constraints on broiler production and is also responsible for inducing high mortality, especially in the finishing phase. Electrolyte balance (EE) and early heat conditioning (CTP) are two techniques that aim to alleviate the negative effects of heat stress. In order to alleviate the effects of heat stress, this study aims to compare early heat conditioning (ETC) and the application of Mongin's principle (electrolyte balance) in the diet. To this end, the electrolyte balance of K+Na-Cl was adjusted to 350 mEq/kg and the electrolyte ratio (K+Cl)/Na to 3:1 using the non-linear PPFR programme (http:// www.fmva.unesp.br/ppfr). The purpose of this study was to evaluate the possible interactions and effects of the electrolyte balance in the diet and the application of early heat conditioning on feed consumption (kg), live weight (kg), feed conversion (kg), mortality (%), bioeconomic energy conversion ratio (Mcal/kg), faecal moisture (%), carcass weight (kg), cavity fat (g) and breast colour (L*a*b*) in broilers under chronic heat stress conditions. To this end, the electrolyte balance (BE = K+Na-Cl) was adjusted to 300 mEq/kg and the electrolyte ratio (RE = [(K+Cl)/Na]) to 3:1 using the non-linear PPFR programme. 640 one-day-old male chicks were housed in a 2x2 factorial arrangement (with and without CTP and with and without EE), in a completely randomised design, in 32 boxes (8 repetitions per treatment). Heat conditioning was carried out on the birds' fifth day of age, for 24 hours at 36 °C, and only on half of the flock (320 birds). After this period, all the birds were transferred to boxes (20 birds/box) with acerola waste as bedding. Chronic heat stress (6 hours at 32°C) was applied to all birds from the 35th to 39th days of age, with the temperature and humidity of the house being monitored electronically in relation to the microclimate of the region/height of the birds. The results indicated that: a) there was no interaction between the two techniques, EE and CTP; b) diets with EE made the feed more expensive and increased the moisture content of the faeces, but there was less mortality; c) CTP resulted in a pale colour in the breast samples. It can therefore be concluded that both EE and CTP are not effective in minimising the negative effects of chronic heat stress in broilers.

Keywords: Formulated feed, electrolytes, chicken, mortality, animal feed, ambient temperature.

CHAPTER 1

INTRODUCTION

Chicken meat stands out on the Brazilian consumer's table because it is a cheap and good quality source of animal protein. According to the Ministry of Agriculture, Brazil has become the world's third largest producer and leading exporter of broiler chicken, and its meat currently reaches 142 countries. The forecast growth rate for chicken meat production is 4.22 per cent per year and exports are expected to grow by 5.62 per cent per year. Brazil should therefore continue to lead the world, but in order to remain at this level, new techniques must be improved to increase poultry productivity in the country (BRASIL, 2015).

As this species is extremely dependent on the ambient temperature for its proper development, birds need different temperature ranges throughout their life cycle. According to recommendations in the Cobb manual (COBB, 2014), from day 0 to day 21 of the bird's life, the temperature of the rearing house should vary between 34 and 24 °C; from day 22 to day 35 of life, the ideal is to maintain the temperature between 24 and 19 °C and, from day 36 to day 42 of life, the temperature of the house should be around 18 °C. Following these recommendations, hot climate regions need practices such as an air-conditioned house, temperature monitoring and a balanced diet to avoid heat stress in the birds.

Heat stress leads to various metabolic disturbances in broiler chickens, including acid-base imbalance. In an attempt to avoid these effects and improve animal performance, it is necessary to use adequate levels of electrolytes and also the correct ratio between them in the feed, i.e. it is necessary to use a formulation with an appropriate electrolyte balance (GAMBA et al., 2015).

Electrolyte balance is basically summarised as electrolyte balance (EB) and electrolyte ratio (ER), where:

"BE = K+Na-CI"   and "RE = (K+CI)/Na"

Since 1981, Mongin (MONGIN, 1981) has proposed the application of electrolyte balance (electrolyte balance and ratio) to mitigate the negative effects of high temperatures on broilers. There has been a great deal of research into the effects of electrolyte balance (AHMAD; SARWAR, 2006), but few studies have fully applied the concepts proposed by Mongin (MINELLO et al., 2012, GAMBA et al., 2015):

a) Meet the minimum requirements for sodium (Na^+), potassium (K^+) and chlorine (Cl^-);
b) Do not present excessive levels;
c) Adjust the balance and electrolyte ratio at the same time.

The only way to fulfil the three requirements imposed by Mongin is through the non-linear formulation. The linear formulation allows the electrolyte balance (Na+K-Cl) to be adjusted, but does not support the adjustment of the electrolyte ratio [(K + Cl)/Na]; but using the non-linear principle of the Practical Programme for Feed Formulation (PPFR) spreadsheet (GARCIA NETO, 2005) it was possible to correctly calculate this type of feed formulation.

In order to meet nutritional demands and keep up with advances in animal genetics, a new mathematical model is required, which is proposed by the non-linear formulation. When you want exact ratios between nutrients, such as Ca and P, or between electrolytes, you need a mathematical device to incorporate a simulator ingredient (PESTI; MILLER, 1992) into the matrix.

For example, when you want Ca/P=2/1, you have Ca=2P, i.e. Ca- 2P=0 (zero). This mathematical manipulation proves to be efficient and is still adopted in linear formulation, but it forces the formulation programme to close the feed at the exact rate, in this case equal to "2". However, with the use of the non-linear principle, as well as simplifying this particular requirement (rates), it makes it possible for them to take on non-specific (fixed) values and so there is no longer any obligation for the ratio to be exactly 2/1 for Ca/P. The same applies to electrolyte balance. In addition, it enables precise formulations without the need to use the inert (SOUZA, 2002), as a substitute for the product under study.

Finally, it should be emphasised that the electrolyte balance of the diet should always be assessed, with concomitant adjustments to the electrolyte balance and ratio, and that this procedure is only possible with the non-linear formulation principle.

In order to assess the possible interactions between two techniques that mitigate the negative effects caused by heat stress, this study evaluated the effects of early heat conditioning (ETC) and electrolyte balance (EE) on broiler performance and carcass characteristics, as well as the economic viability of adopting these strategies to minimise the effects of an adverse thermal environment.

CHAPTER 2

LITERATURE REVIEW

2.1 Thermal stress

Brazil, a country with a tropical climate, has, among its many challenges in poultry farming, the environmental factor - high temperature and high humidity inside the house - as a limiting factor for optimum productivity, since high temperatures reduce food consumption and harm the performance of the chickens (FURLAN, 2006).

Thus, various metabolic and physiological changes are triggered in broilers subjected to high environmental temperatures, which can lead to major losses in the performance and immunocompetence of these birds (BORGES et al., 2003).

However, some measures can be taken to minimise losses due to heat stress, including the use of fans and nebulisers, manipulation of protein and energy levels in the diet, acclimatising the birds, the use of antipyretics, ascorbic acid and electrolytes, feed management and drinking water management (BORGES, 1997).

Above 30°C, feed consumption decreases rapidly and energy requirements increase due to the birds' need to eliminate heat. Therefore, this lower feed consumption and energy expenditure to maintain thermal homeostasis leads to a reduction in the performance of birds reared at high temperatures (FURLAN, 2006).

Among the compensatory physiological responses of birds when exposed to heat is peripheral vasodilation, resulting in an increase in non-evaporative heat loss. In an attempt to increase heat dissipation, the bird increases its surface area by keeping its wings away from its body, ruffling its feathers and intensifying peripheral circulation (BORGES et al., 2003).

Non-evaporative heat loss can also occur with increased urine production, if this water loss is compensated for by increased cold water consumption. Another physiological response is the increase in respiration rate, evaporative heat loss, resulting in excessive losses of carbon dioxide (CO_2). Thus, the partial pressure of CO_2 (pCO_2) decreases, leading to a drop in the concentration of carbonic acid (H_2CO_3) and hydrogen (H+). In response, the kidneys increase the excretion of bicarbonate (HCO_3)

and reduce the excretion of H^+ in an attempt to maintain the bird's acid-base balance. This change in acid-base balance is known as respiratory alkalosis and can lead to high bird mortality (BORGES et al., 2003).

In order to mitigate this effect in broiler chickens in the growth phase and, especially, close to finishing, as they are more sensitive to high temperatures, various investigations into thermoregulation have been carried out (GAMBA et al., 2015; MINELLO et al., 2012; VIEIRA, 2008; YAHAV; HURWITZ, 1996; YAHAV; McMURTRY, 2001). A very strong reason for the need for this knowledge is that maintaining the ideal temperature between 18 and 20°C in tropical countries is economically unfeasible. As a consequence, there are losses in performance and, depending on the situation, increased mortality in broiler chickens (RUTZ, 1994).

2.2 Electrolyte balance

The need for balance is vital for every living being, both the balance of the external environment (air, water, temperature, humidity, food) and the balance of the internal environment (cells, metabolic functions, body fluids).

With regard to the environmental factor, the environment of a broiler house must be managed so as not to compromise the narrow limits of the various physiological processes of the birds, i.e. the maintenance of homeostasis, which is basically the maintenance of the composition of the internal environment compatible with the survival of individual cells. The attempt to maintain this balance takes place mainly in a tropical country like Brazil, where high temperatures and humidity rates are constant challenges to the zootechnical performance of poultry (FURLAN, 2006).

According to Mongin (1981), in order to maintain acid-base homeostasis in equilibrium, an animal needs to have a cationic dietary intake plus endogenous acid production (H^+) minus the cationic difference excreted, equal to zero. Of these combinations (ingested + endogenous - excreted), the one that is easiest to control is the proportion of minerals in the diet, as it is directly related to the plasma concentration of bicarbonate (HCO_3^-) (MONGIN; SAUVEUR,1977).

The minerals K^+ , Na^+ and Cl^- , in particular, are chosen because of their importance in metabolism, their participation in the osmotic balance, the acid-base balance and the integrity of the mechanisms that regulate transport across cell membranes. Thus, these minerals act directly on the acid-base balance of poultry and can jeopardise performance by compromising many metabolic functions (JUDICE et al., 2002).

As electrolytes are responsible for maintaining body water and the ionic balance, the ideal concentration of Na^+ , K^+ and Cl^- cannot be determined independently, due to the interactions between these ions in the diet and subsequently in the birds' metabolism (COHEN et al., 1972; JUNQUEIRA et al.,1984; NOBAKHT et al., 2006).

This highlights the importance of a feed having a favourable electrolyte balance, but there are still doubts about how best to adapt a diet to this new concept, whether by difference (Na+K-Cl), ratios (K + Cl)/Na or (K+Na)/Cl or both (difference and ratio), as well as defining the most appropriate values according to the stage of rearing (BORGATTI et al., 2004).

Plasma Na+, K+ and Cl- levels are affected by heat stress. K+ and Na+ concentrations decrease as temperature increases (BORGES et al., 1999), while Cl- increases (BELAY; TEETER, 1993).

According to Mongin (1981), the acid-base balance of the diet for Na^+ , K^+ and Cl^- , previously formulated only to meet the minimum requirement for each stage of rearing (NRC, 1994), should have its proportions adjusted for a better electrolyte balance (EB), aiming for optimum growth performance by maintaining the animal's physiological acid-base homeostasis (GEZEN et al., 2005).

Recently, several studies have been aimed at developing simplified electrolyte balance expressions in order to identify critical values and the most appropriate relationship between electrolytes for use and application in the feeding of various species (HAYDON; WEST, 1990; ROSS et al. 1994; WILDMAN et al., 2007).

Therefore, for an adequate electrolyte balance of a diet, it would not be enough just to calculate the difference between the total concentration of anions and cations, but also the appropriate proportion between K and Na (LEWIS et al., 1972; TALBOT, 1978).

For broilers, the ideal level of variation is around 250 mEq/kg or 25 mEq/100g (BORGES, 2006), as described by the simplified formula $[Na^+] + [K^+] - [Cl^-]$ (MONGIN, 1981; JOHNSON; KARUNAJEEWA, 1985; VIEITES et al., 2004; VIEITES et al., 2005).

According to Gamba et al. (2015), it was possible to verify that the strategic use of non-linear formulation with the correct electrolyte balance improves performance and is able to avoid the effect of heat stress in broilers, considering a diet with BE of 250 mEq/kg and RE 3, for better performance in thermoneutral conditions, and a diet with BE of 350 mEq/kg and RE 3 aimed at the survival of the animals in conditions of heat stress.

The addition and manipulation of electrolytes such as sodium bicarbonate ($NaHCO_3$), potassium chloride (KCl), calcium chloride ($CaCl_2$) and ammonium chloride (NH_4Cl) in water or feed minimises the effects of heat stress on birds (BORGES et al., 1999; SOUZA et al., 2002; BORGES et al., 2003), bringing slaughter forward by two days during the summer, as well as favouring feed conversion and reducing mortality (BENTON et al., 1998).

In this sense, the electrolyte balance helps to maintain the acid-base balance in order to minimise the birds' predisposition to respiratory alkalosis as a result of heat stress and, consequently, its negative effects on weight gain (TEETER et al., 1985), 1985) caused by lower food intake and poorer feed conversion, as well as the incidence of PSE (pale, soft and exudative) meat in poultry (WOELFEL et al., 2002; MOREIRA, 2005), which is not preferred by consumers (TAKAHASHI, 2007).

With knowledge of the impact of the acid-base balance on animal production, nutritionists must pay greater attention to diet formulation, due to its influence on feed consumption and bird development (RIDDELL, 1975; PATICIENCE et al., 1987; BORGATTI et al., 2004), health (SAVEUR, 1984), the expression of the animals' genetic potential (THORP et al., 1993; FURLAN, 2006), 1993), as well as responses to heat stress (TEERTER et al., 1985; FURLAN, 2006), in addition to their interference in the metabolism of amino acids (HARA et al., 1987), minerals (LUTZ, 1984) and vitamins (REDDY et al., 1982; THORP et al., 1993), which demonstrates the need for a greater understanding of these interactions (PESTI et al., 1991; PATIENCE, 1990; BORGATTI et al., 2004).

The current concern of nutritionists is to establish the balance of the diet for the supply of cations and anions (LEESON et al., 1995), since the manipulation of electrolytes in the diet is simple, practical and economical, and the requirements for Na, K and Cl are already clearly defined (NRC, 1994);
ROSTAGNO et al., 2011). According to Leeson et al. (1995), the electrolyte balance can affect the metabolism of various amino acids, especially lysine and arginine. Therefore, there is a need to know and understand these interactions better, in order to obtain feed formulations with better nutritional adjustments and thus avoid metabolic disorders triggered by the acid-base imbalance of poultry diets (COELLO et al., 2008).

2.3 Early thermal conditioning (ETC)

Birds can be physiologically manipulated to better tolerate heat stress through acclimatisation or heat conditioning. Acclimatisation allows for better thermotolerance, but has the disadvantage of impairing bird performance. Thermal conditioning, on the other hand, is more favourable, allowing for a better response to thermotolerance, as it does not adversely affect the birds' final performance. However, it is dependent on compensatory gain (YAHAV; McMURTRY, 2001; VIEIRA, 2008).

Currently, heat acclimatisation is the best known aspect of broiler production. It consists of rearing the birds at a temperature above the thermoneutral range during the initial and growth phases, resulting in their adaptation to the heat and, consequently, a lower mortality rate due to heat stress in the finishing phase (VIEIRA, 2008).

However, chickens acclimatised to heat show a reduction in final weight gain due to lower food consumption and greater energy expenditure to maintain metabolic activities. Due to these limitations, the early heat conditioning (EHT) technique emerged, in which birds are exposed to extreme temperatures (35 to 38°C) for around 24 hours at a time during the initial rearing phase (between the third and fifth day of age) (VIEIRA, 2008).

A possible mechanism for the acquisition of thermal tolerance is the ability to reduce heat production, which is regulated to a large extent by the hormone Triiodothyronine (T3), the concentration of which is reduced at high temperatures. Thus, it can be predicted that the induction of thermotolerance by temperature conditioning is associated with the modulation of T3 concentration in the plasma (YAHAV; HURWITZ, 1996).

CHAPTER 3

HYPOTHESIS

The following hypothesis was raised:

Electrolyte balance, applied in conjunction with heat conditioning, minimises the undesirable effects of heat stress in broilers.

CHAPTER 4

OBJECTIVES

The purpose of this project was to evaluate the possible interactions and effects of electrolyte balance in the diet and the application of early heat conditioning on feed consumption (kg), live weight (kg), feed conversion (kg), mortality (%), bioeconomic energy index (Mcal/kg), faeces moisture (%), carcass weight (kg), cavity fat (g) and breast colour (L*a*b*) in broilers under chronic heat stress conditions.

CHAPTER 5

MATERIAL AND METHODS

5.1 Treatments and experimental design

The experimental rations (Table 1) were called traditional rations (without EE) and rations with electrolyte balance (starter ration: BE = 250 mEq/kg and RE = 3:1 and growth and finishing rations: BE = 300 mEq/kg and RE = 3:1).

°Table 1 - Composition and cost of starter (1st to 21st day), grower (22nd to 35th day) and finisher (36th to 42nd day) rations used in the experiment to feed the birds

Nutrient	Unit -	Calculated composition					
		Traditional feed			Feed with EE		
		Home	Growth	Termination	Home	Growth	Termination
Cost of feed	Rl/100 kg	76,81	74,53	67,15	78,53	78,37	71,49
Energy Met. Poultry	kcal/kg	2980,00	3050,00	3100,00	2980,00	3050,00	3100,00
Crude Protein (CP)	%	20,62	19,14	17,84	20,66	19,13	17,83
Calcium	%	0,86	0,75	0,65	0,86	0,75	0,65
P Available	%	0,38	0,34	0,29	0,38	0,34	0,29
Potassium	%	0,81	0,75	0,69	0,85	0,98	0,97
Sodium	%	0,21	0,20	0,20	0,21	0,23	0,23
Chlorine	%	0,38	0,36	0,36	0,20	0,18	0,17
Linoleic acid	%	2,52	2,69	2,61	2,60	2,91	2,87
Dig.	%	1,14	1,05	0,97	1,14	1,05	0,97
Methionine Dig.	%	0,54	0,50	0,46	0,54	0,50	0,46
Methionine + Cystine Dig.	%	0,82	0,76	0,71	0,82	0,76	0,71
Threonine Dig.	%	0,74	0,68	0,63	0,74	0,68	0,63
Tryptophan Dig.	%	0,23	0,21	0,19	0,23	0,21	0,19
BE- K+Na -Cl (mEq/kg)*	mEq	191,70	176,27	160,94	250,00	300,00	300,00
RE= (K+Cl)/Na*	-	3,42	3,36	3,27	3,00	3,00	3,00
		Ingredients					
Maize (7.88%)	%	59,32	63,44	68,02	58,79	62,07	66,45
Soya meal (45%)	%	34,68	30,74	26,98	34,86	30,97	27,24
Soya oil	%	2,06	2,30	2,04	2,22	2,77	2,58
Bicalcium phosphate	%	1.47	1,24	1,03	1,47	1,24	1,03
Calcitic limestone	%	1,06	0,94	0,83	1,06	0,94	0,83
Polimax F**	%	0,60	0,60	0,30	0,60	0,60	0,30
Sodium Bicarbonate	%	0,00	0,00	0,00	0,41	0,55	0,57
Common Salt	%	0,48	0,46	0,44	0,20	0,16	0,13
L-Lysine HCl	%	0,18	0,18	0,20	0,18	0,18	0,19
DL-Methionine	%	0,11	0,08	0,14	0,11	0,09	0,14
Potassium carbonate 99.5%	%	0,00	0,00	0,00	0,07	0,42	0,51
L-Threonine	%	0,04	0,03	0,02	0,04	0,03	0,02

*BE - electrolyte balance; RE = electrolyte ratio

"A Composition of vitamin-mineral supplements used in feed during the three rearing phases (quantity/kg of product): Initial: vit A - 1,670,000 U.I; vit. D3- 335,000 U.I; vit. E -2,500 mg; vit K3- 417 mg; vit B1 - 250 mg; vit. B2- 835 mg; vit. B6 - 250 mg; vit. B12 - 2,000 mcg; folic acid - 100 mg, biotin - 9 mg; niacin - 5,835 mg; calcium pantothenate - 1.870 mg; Cu 1,000 mg; Co 17 mg; I 170 mg; Fe 8,335 mg; Mn - 10,835mg; Zn - 7,500 mg; Se - 35 mg; Choline Chloride 50% 116,670 mg; Methionine - 250,000 mg; Coceidiostatic -13,335 mg; Growth Promoter - 13,335 mg; Antioxidant - 2,000 mg. Growth: vit A -1,335,000 U.I; vit. D3-300,000 U.I; vit. E -2,000 mg; vit. K3 -335 mg; vit B1 -167 mg; vit B2- 670 mg; vit. B6 -170 mg; vit. B12 -1,670 mcg; folic acid - 67 mg; biotin -7 mg; niacin - 4,670 mg; calcium pantothenate - 1.870 mg; Cu - 1,000 mg; Co - 17 mg I -170 mg; Fe - 8,335 mg; Mn - 10,835 mg; Zn - 7,500 mg; Se - 35 mg; Choline Chloride 50% - 83,340mg; Methionine - 235,000mg; Coccidiostat - 10,000 mg; Growth Promoter - 10,000mg; Antioxidant - 2,000mg. Finishing: vit A - 1,670,000 U.I; vit D3 - 335,000 U.I; vit E - 2,335 mg; vit K3 - 400 mg; vit B1 -100 mg; vit B2 - 800 mg; vit B6 - 200 mg; vit B12 - 2,000 mcg; folic acid - 67 mg; biotin - 7 mg; niacin - 5,670 mg; calcium pantothenate - 2.000 mg; Cu - 2,000 mg; Co - 27 mg; I - 270 mg; Fe - 16,670 mg, Mn - 17,335 mg; Zn - 12,000 mg; Se - 70 mg; Choline Chloride 50% - 100,000mg; Methionine - 235,000mg, Antioxidant - 2,000 mg Dosage of 6kg of product per tonne of feed.

The treatments were labelled A, B, C and D, according to whether or not they combined electrolyte balance in the diet and early heat conditioning (Table 2).

Table 2 - Treatment according to the combination of the application or not of electrolyte balance in the diets and early heat conditioning of broilers

Treatment	EE application [1]	Conditioning application early thermal
A	No	No
B	Yes	Yes
C	No	Yes
D	Yes	No

Electrolyte balance {EEfelectrolyte balance/mEq/kg)=(Na/22.99 + K/39 10 - Cl/35.45)*1000 and RE[electrolyte ratio=(K/39 10 + Cl/35.45)/(Na/22.99)]}. [2]
Early heat conditioning (application at 5 days of age of the birds, for 24 hours, of 36ʳ C).

The experiment was a completely randomised design, in a 2x2 factorial arrangement (with and without TCP and with and without EE), totalling 4 treatments, with eight replications and 20 birds per experimental plot (total 640 birds), whose analysis of variance scheme is shown in Table 3.

Table 3 Analysis of variance model for the experiment

Sources of Variation	Degrees of Freedom
Electrolytic balance (EE)	1
Early thermal conditioning (ETC)	1
EE x CTP	1
Error	28
Total	31

5.2 Conducting the experiment

The experiment was carried out in the Experimental Zootechnics Sector of the Veterinary Medicine Course at UNESP, Araçatuba Campus. 640 male broiler chicks of the same commercial strain (Cobb 500) were used from 1 to 42 days of age.

The birds (1-6 days old) were housed in metal cages and then in a masonry shed (7.85 x 45.70 metres), facing east-west, air-conditioned with an adiabatic evaporative cooling system with negative pressure ventilation, covered with special tiles made of insulating material (expanded polystyrene) sandwiched between reflective metal sheets.

After being housed in batteries, the birds were placed in boxes (7-42 days old) measuring 1.4 x 3.0 metres, which formed the experimental plots, with acerola waste as the floor.

The one-day-old chicks were weighed and randomly assigned to metal cages with 20 birds each. 60 W lamps (batteries) were used as initial heating sources, one in each compartment, with automated heating adjustment. The birds subjected to CTP on the 5th day of life (half the batch, 320 birds) remained in the cages and the rest were placed in their respective boxes.

After this period, all the birds went into the boxes, where they were heated using porcelain cones with 400 W resistance installed in hoods.

The experimental rations were mixed at the Zootechnics Experimental Sector's feed mill and were based on corn, soya meal, oil, vitamin supplement, mineral supplement, limestone and bicalcium phosphate (Table 1), following the recommendations of Rostagno et al. (2011), and the salts sodium chloride (NaCl), sodium bicarbonate ($NaHCO_3$) and potassium carbonate (K_2CO_3) were added according to the minimum Na, K and Cl requirements and the electrolyte adjustments required for each experimental feed, using the non-linear PPFR programme for broilers (GARCIA NETO, 2005).

The birds were subjected to chronic heat stress (GONZALEZ- ESQUERRA; LEESON, 2006), with an average temperature of 32°C for a period of 6 hours, from the 35th to the 39th day of age (Figure 1). For this to be possible, the barn's cooling system was switched off and the heating system was set to a maximum of 32.5°C.

Days 1 2 3 4 5 6 7 8 9 10 11 12 13 14 15 16 17 18 19 20 21 22 23 24 25 26 27 28 29 30 31 32 33 34 35 36 37 38 39 40 41 42
Condicionamento Térmico Precoce (36°C por 24 h), apenas em metade do lote (320 aves).
32 Boxes de 1.5 x 3m (20 aves/boxe). Cama de semente de acerola.
Aves expostas ao Estresse Térmico Crônico (32°C) - 6 h por dia do 35º ao 39º dias de idade, em todos os tratamentos.

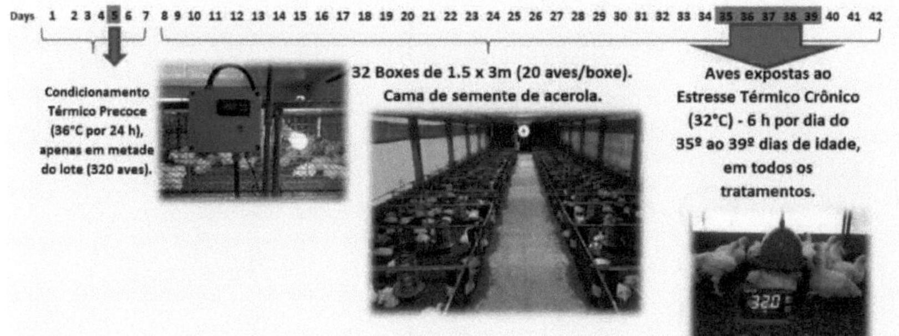

FIGURE 1 - Summary of the experiment - Application of early heat conditioning and chronic heat stress.

Air temperature and humidity measurements were taken using *ibutons* **installed inside** white **polyvinyl chloride** (PVC) **"T" fittings** and black globes (Figure 2). The *ibutons* **in the "T" fittings** took readings every 20 minutes and the globes every 10 minutes. Subsequently, the average temperature of the house for each day was calculated. The sensors were installed in the shade, at bird height, every 2 boxes, as shown in Figure 3.

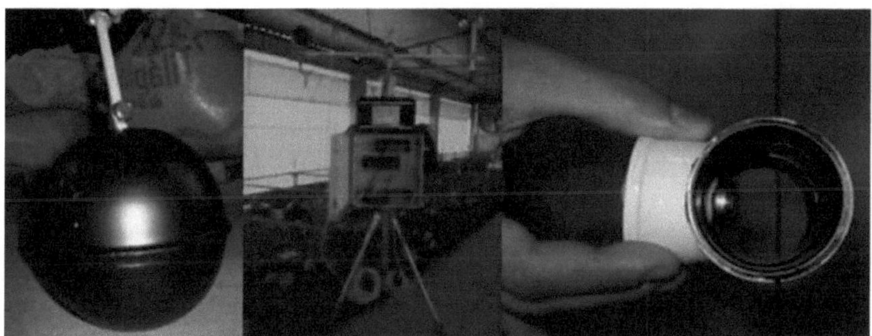

FIGURE 2 - Equipment for controlling and characterising temperature and humidity in the shed. On the left - black globe thermometer; in the middle - automatic weather station, on the right - *Ibuttori®*.

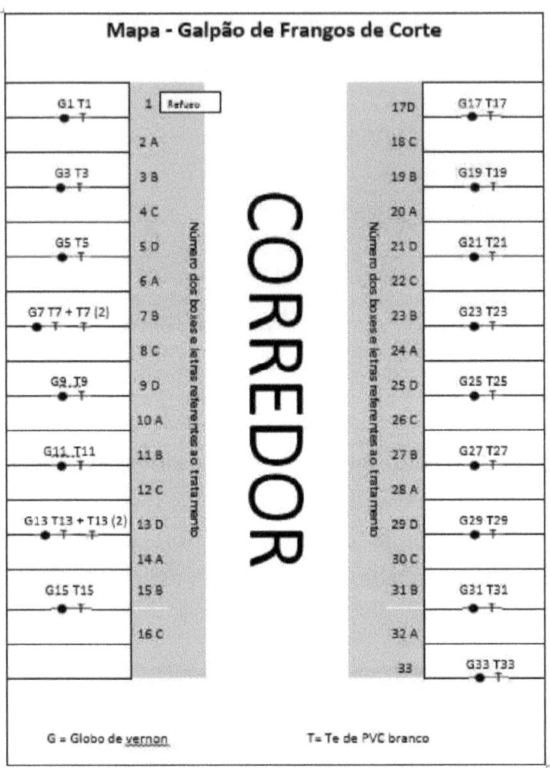

FIGURE 3 - Sketch of the experimental shed with the distribution of treatments (A, B, C and D) and the installation of the black globes and "Ts" with *ibutons*.

5. 3Evaluations

5.3. 1Bird performance

The birds were assessed on the 21st and 42nd days of age for corrected feed consumption (g/bird/period), corrected feed conversion and weight gain (g/bird/period). The birds were observed twice a day (morning and afternoon), and any mortality was recorded on the corrected feed consumption and feed conversion spreadsheet (APPENDIX B).

5.3. 2Economic index

The economic viability of each treatment was calculated using the Bioeconomic Energy Conversion (BEC) index (GARCIA NETO et al., 2012). However, for this experiment, the formula was improved (Figure 4) and the BEC spreadsheet was developed (APPENDIX C).

$$BEC = \frac{[(a1*b1*c1)+(a2*b2*c2)+(a3*b3*c3)]}{(d*e)} = Mcal/kg$$

Where:

a1= Initial feed intake (kg) a2= Growth feed consumption (kg) a3= Finishing feed consumption (kg)
b1 = Initial feed cost (R$/kg) b2 = Cost of growth feed (R$/kg) b3 = Cost of finishing feed (R$/kg)
c1 = Metabolisable energy of starter feed (Mcal/kg) c2 = Metabolisable energy of growth feed (Mcal/kg) c3 = Metabolisable energy of finishing feed (Mcal/kg) d = Final weight of live batch (kg)
e = Price paid per kg of live chicken (R$)

FIGURE 4 - Improved BEC index formula.

5.3.3 Carcass yield and colour analysis

The weight of abdominal fat and the weight of each carcass of 3 birds with a live weight similar to the average weight of each repetition, totalling 96 birds, were determined at 42 days of age.

In the frozen carcass, 24 hours after slaughter, colour analysis was carried out on boneless, skinless breast samples kept at 4°C (WOELFEL et al., 2002). To do this, a Mini Scan XE Plus portable reflected colour spectrophotometer (HunterLab) was used, calibrated with black and white standards and expressed according to the CIE L*a*b* colour system of the Comission Internationale de l'Eclairage. The L* value represents clarity, ranging from zero, which means there is no clarity (absolute black) to 100, which is maximum clarity (absolute white). The a* value varies from green (negative values) to red (positive values) and the b* value varies from blue (negative values) to yellow (positive values) (MINOLTA, 2007).

5.3.4 Moisture in faeces

Excreta samples were collected on the 42nd day of each experimental plot to assess humidity. The 32 samples were pre-dried in an oven at 55°C for 72 hours and then dried in an oven at 105°C for 12 hours, according to the methodology proposed by Silva and Queiroz (2002).

5. 4Statistical analysis

The results were analysed to check for treatment effects and to assess the effects of each factor, using the PROC GLM procedures in the SAS system (2009). Student's t-test was used to check the significance of differences between treatment means.

CHAPTER 6

RESULTS AND DISCUSSION

The results of the performance, mortality, economic index (BEC) and faecal moisture of the broilers subjected to the different treatments are shown in Table 4.

Table *i* - Effects of the combination of early heat conditioning (ETC) and electrolytic equilibrium (EE), associated with the application of chronic heat stress in birds aged 35 to 39 days, on the averages for feed consumption, live weight, feed conversion, mortality, bioeconomic energy conversion (BEC) and faecal moisture of male broilers aged 1-42 days.

	Feed consumption (kg)		Live weight (kg)		Feed conversion		Mortality (%)	BEC	Moisture in
Factors	1-21 days	1-42 days	21 days	42 dayo	21 days	42 days	1-42 days	(Mcal/kg)	Faeces (%)
With CTP	1,24	5,02	0,92	3,14	1,36	1,60	3,06	1,69	80,46
Without CTP	1,21	4,93	0,91	3,15	1,33	1,56	3,06	1,66	81,63
With EE	1,24	5,00	0,93	3,16	1,34	1,58	2,44 (100*)	1,71 (104) A	82,14 (103) A
No EE	1,21	4,95	0,90	3,13	1,35	1,58	3,69 (151)	1,64 (100*) B	79,95 (100*) B
Sources of variation	Pr> F	Pr> F	Pr> F	Pr> F	Pr > F	Pr > F	Pr> F	Pr> F	Pr> F
CTP	0,3048	0,2585	0,9487	0,7850	0,3880	0,0963	0,9922	0,942	0,1694
EE	0,3146	0,5313	0,2704	0,4370	0,7588	0,8807	0,1154	0,0037	0,0134
CTP x EE	0,4706	0,4293	0,2864	0,8080	0,6224	0,421	0,4696	0,4048	0,1257
CV(%)	4,97	4,54	7,24	2,90	6,60	3,51	5,43	3,52	2,91

Averages followed by the same letter in the columns do not differ statistically by the T-test (P>0.05).

BEC=(feed consumption*feed cost*metabolisable energy)/(kg weight gain*kg live chicken price). * Relative value (%)

No interaction effects were found for any of the parameters evaluated. This means that there was no synergism when CTP and the electrolyte balance (EE) diet were applied simultaneously.

The assessment of bird performance showed no statistical difference, with p > 0.05. Similarly, statistically, there was no difference in terms of mortality, however, according to Haaland (1989 apud RODRIGUES; IEMMA, 2009), when there is a p < 0.1 it is necessary to pay more attention to this variable.

> When selecting variables, it is probably better to accept a p-value of <0.1 than to leave an important factor out. The researcher's practical judgement should be the final arbiter. Use common sense when interpreting statistical analyses. Beware of the syndrome: *"STATISTICS ON, BRAIN OFF.* (HAALAND, 1989 apud RODRIGUES; IEMMA, 2009, p. 174.

According to Table 4, mortality, with a p-value of 0.1154, averaged 2.44 per cent in the EE treatments, while diets without EE had a mortality rate of 3.69 per cent. Thus, it can be concluded that diets without EE increased the average mortality of thermally stressed birds by 51%. Gamba et al. (2015) reached the same conclusion in their experiment, stating that formulating feed with an adequate electrolyte balance led to greater survival of thermally stressed birds. Similarly, BENTON et al. (1998) found a reduction in mortality in birds that received added electrolytes and were exposed to heat.

Despite this, EE is unfavourable for broilers when subjected to chronic stress, in bioeconomic terms, making the feed more expensive and also because it favours wetter faeces (Table 4). The rations became more expensive because they tried to accommodate the principle of electrolyte balance in the formulation.

With the addition of the electrolytes potassium carbonate (K_2CO_3) and sodium bicarbonate ($NaHCO_3$) to fulfil the electrolyte balance proposed in this experiment, there was an increase in feed cost and a worse BEC value (the higher the value, the lower the cost benefit of the treatment). According to Oliveira et al. (2004), one option would be to reduce the BE value, as in their experiment with pigs, changing the BE value from 210 to 170 mEq/kg reduced feed costs without interfering with performance.

The economic evaluation of animal nutritional performance is necessary to verify the real profit margin in a production. The BEC differs in that it incorporates the most expensive item in a diet (energy), making it more efficient and coherent in representing costs/benefits, by measuring energy consumption in terms of bioeconomic conversion, i.e. the best performance and, energetically, the greatest economic return, with the result that the lower the index, the better the cost/benefit.

Another negative factor for diets formulated with the proposed EE was the increase in excreta humidity (Table 4), since it resulted in pastier excreta, with 82.14% humidity, which is known to favour litter impairment, since it absorbs humidity, which under normal conditions is around 80% (AVILA et al., 1992) in wood shavings. It is plausible that this increase is mainly due to the higher potassium content of the diet (Table 1, Figures 5 and 6).

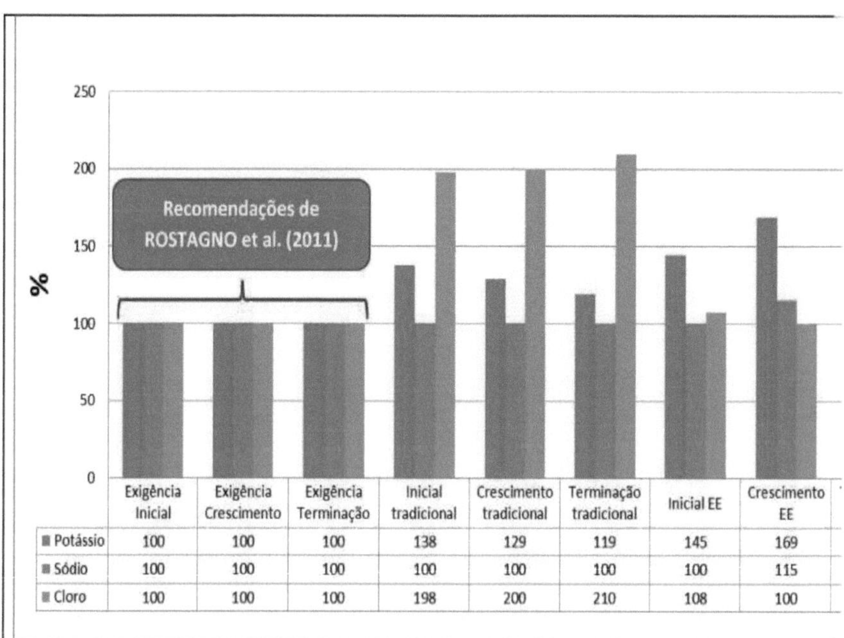

	Exigência Inicial	Exigência Crescimento	Exigência Terminação	Inicial tradicional	Crescimento tradicional	Terminação tradicional	Inicial EE	Crescimento EE
Potássio	100	100	100	138	129	119	145	169
Sódio	100	100	100	100	100	100	100	115
Cloro	100	100	100	198	200	210	108	100

Figure 5 Comparative graphs between the minimum recommendations (index 100) and the principles of traditional formulation and electrolyte balance (EE).

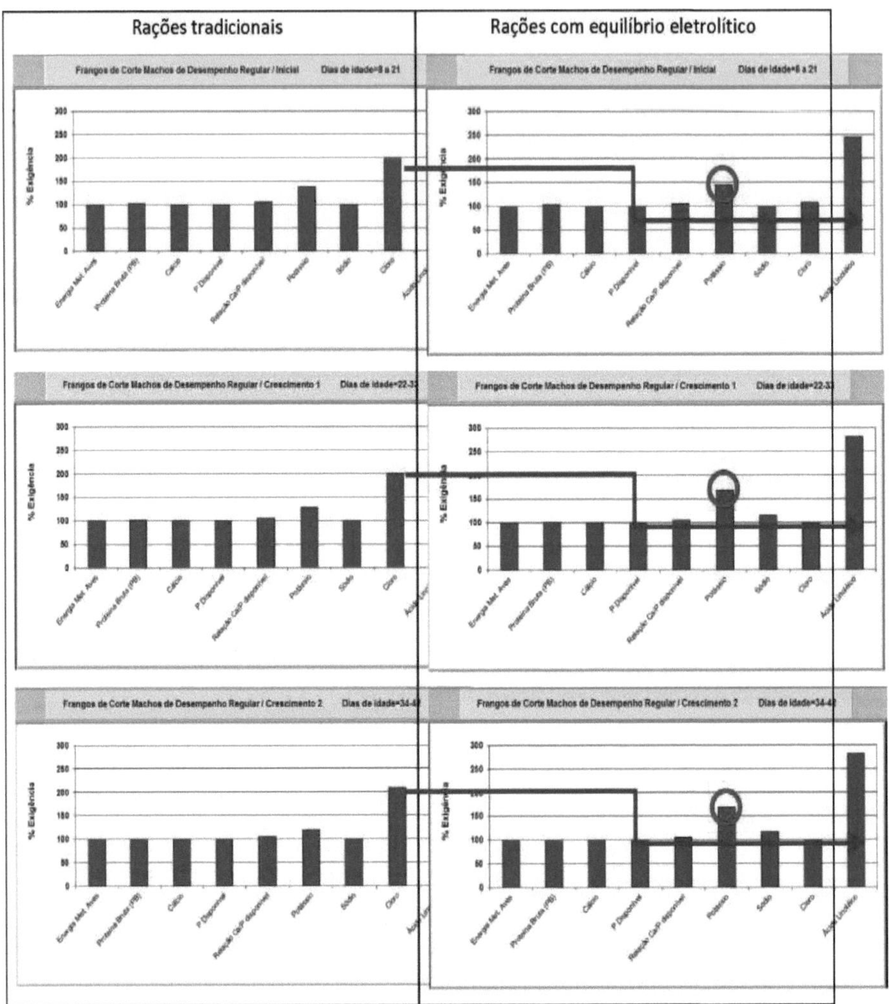

Figure 6: Percentage requirements of nutrients in the diet, according to phase and formulation principle (Traditional vs. Electrolyte balance)

According to Casado and Virseda (1983) and Oliveira et al. (2003), both Na+ and K+ supplementation increase water excretion. Excess Na+ increases water consumption and excess K+ results in greater urinary loss (ARAÚJO et al., 2010). Consequently, both result in an increase in litter moisture due to pastier faeces.

Several studies have confirmed that adding potassium (KCl) to drinking water or feed favours increased water consumption by broilers reared in conditions of heat

stress (BORGES, 1999). For this reason, it is
It is common to recommend the use of feed additives to increase water consumption in conditions of heat stress, with the aim of helping broiler chickens' body heat loss mechanisms (SMITH; TEETER, 1987; BORGES,1999; SOUZA, 2002).

However, when the amount of water ingested increases, the volume excreted also rises proportionally, affecting litter quality due to increased faecal moisture (MACARI, 1996), which is detrimental to bird management and development (GAMBA et al., 2015). Thus, the increase in faecal moisture is due to excess Na^+ , excess K^+ and heat stress, because according to Barbosa Filho (2004), water consumption can be up to 0.5 litres/bird/day, with temperatures above the thermal comfort range (18 to 20°C) of the birds.

Increased water intake by chickens can be beneficial in conditions of heat stress (TEETER et al., 1985; MACARI et al., 1994), but this benefit was not found in the birds subjected to chronic stress in the present experiment.

The increase in potassium levels is due to two reasons: 1) the main source of protein used for this formulation is soya meal, which has a high level of potassium in its composition (ARAÚJO et al., 2010; ROSTAGNO, 2011); and 2) the use of potassium carbonate to formulate the experimental diets with electrolyte balance (BE = 300 mEq/kg and RE = 3).

This was not the case with the starter, as the requirement was set at BE = 250 mEq/kg. Therefore, for better formulation adjustments, it would be advisable to use an electrolyte balance of between 250 and 300 mEq/kg and an electrolyte ratio of between 2 and 3. However, the formulation in this experiment followed the recommendations of Gamba et al. (2015), aiming for an electrolyte balance that offered better performance (BE = 250 mEq/kg) adjusted to greater survival (BE = 350 mEq/kg) under conditions of heat stress.

Another option for adjusting the formulation would be to opt for another protein source for the diet, with a lower concentration of potassium levels.

Excess potassium in the feed jeopardises the quality and useful life of the litter. This emphasises the need to formulate balanced diets for broilers. Birds are more tolerant of excess K^+ than Na^+ (SAVEUR; MONGIN, 1978), but excess Na^+ is easily corrected and does not interfere with the birds' development (GAMBA et al., 2015).

However, diets formulated with high levels of Cl- (NH_4Cl, IICl, NaCl and $CaCl_2$) lower the blood pH in chickens, jeopardising their growth in thermoneutral conditions. According to Gamba et al. (2015), birds performed better when fed diets with lower Cl concentrations.

The results for the statistical analyses of carcass weight, cavity fat weight and colour attributes for males, according to each treatment, are shown in Table 5.

Table 5 - Effects of the combination of early heat conditioning (ETC) and electrolytic equilibrium (EE), associated with the application of chronic heat stress in birds from 35 to 39 days of age, on the averages for carcass weight without feet and head, cavity fat and breast colour characteristic (L*a*b*) of male broilers from 1-42 days of age

Factors	Weight Carcass (kg)	Cavity fat (g)	Breast colour L*	a*	b*
With CTP	2,61	0,056	58,82 A	7,93	18,06 A
i Without CTP	2,62	0,053	56,25 B	8,19	17,22B
ComEE	2,61	0,054	58,31	7,96	17,78
No EE	2,62	0,055	56,77	8,17	17,50
Sources of variation	Pr>F	Pr>F	Pr>F	Pr>F	Pr>F
CTP	0,6954	0,4184	0,0123	0,4375	0,048
EE	0,8329	0,6844	0,1213	0,5249	0,5052
CTP x EE	0,1818	0,4184	0,1196	0,7900	0,7122
CV(%)	4,44	15,83	4,72	11,58	6,56

Averages followed by the same letter in the columns do not differ statistically by the T-test (P>0.05) L*=Luminosity expressed as a percentage (from 0 for black and 100 for white): a*=red/green coordinate (+a indicates red and -a indicates green); b'=yellow/blue coordinate (+b indicates yellow and -b indicates blue) - Available at: htt0://sensing.konicaminolta.com.br/2013/11/entendendo-o-espaco- d e -c o r-1 a b/#st h a s h 5fVQ kP AX. d puf.

Also, for the variables carcass weight (kg); cavity fat weight (g) and breast colour (L*a*b*), there were no significant interactions between the factors studied, showing the independent action of these attributes.

Significant differences were only found for the colour attributes L* and b* (L* values as measures of whiteness, a* for reddish and b* for yellowish).

Breast colour was lighter or paler and more yellowish for those birds subjected to CTP, i.e. the birds with the longest exposure to heat stress in life, on the fifth day of heat conditioning and again from the 35th to 39th days, when challenged to a period of chronic heat stress (Figure 7).

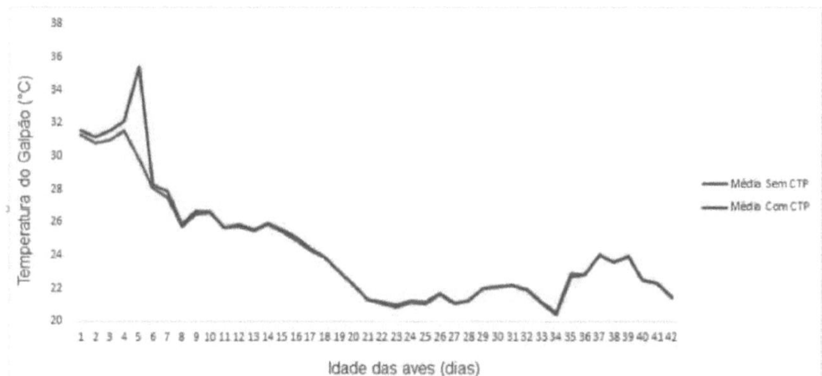

Figure 7. Average house temperature according to the age of the birds. Application of early heat conditioning on day 5 (24 h at 36 °C) and chronic heat stress from day 35 to 39 (6 h per day at 32 °C).

Similarly, Bianchi et al. (2007) found higher L* and b* values in broiler breasts slaughtered during the summer. Heat stress immediately before slaughter has been shown to affect the colour of turkey meat (NGOKA; FRONING, 1982) and broiler meat (NORTHCUTT et al., 1994). In part, the present experiment confirms that heat stress can compromise broiler presentation in terms of colour (Table 5).

All the L* values in this experiment were above 49 and according to Takahashi (2007) the L* value greater than or equal to 49 is used to indicate the occurrence of pale meat, considering this parameter to be representative of changes in meat quality characteristics.

As well as affecting the colour of the carcass, the L* value is also related to the water retention capacity of the carcass. In other words, the higher the L* value, the lower the water retention capacity, and the breast will have a less tender texture. Therefore, a high L* value is not a good standard for broiler carcasses, as not only does it result in less tender meat, but it also alters the colour, making it look paler, which is not to the consumer's liking (TAKAHASHI, 2007).

The expectation that heat-stressed chickens would deposit more fat in the carcass (CHENG et al., 1997) was not confirmed in this experiment.

In view of the results obtained, both early heat conditioning and electrolyte balance in the diet were not effective in minimising the negative effects caused by chronic heat stress in broilers. This result is compatible with that found by Vieira (2008), who concluded that CTP was unable to induce a degree of adaptation to heat sufficient to improve the productive and carcass characteristics of chickens subjected to chronic stress.

However, the literature shows good results from these strategies for acute stress, according to Yahav and McMurtry (2001), Minello et al. (2012) and Gamba, et al. (2015).

However, further research is needed into CTP and EE techniques for broilers under high temperatures (acute and chronic stress) and with other ratio values and electrolyte balance.

CHAPTER 7

CONCLUSIONS

1- There was no interaction effect with the application of early heat conditioning (EHT) simultaneously with electrolyte balance (EE). However, EE is unfavourable for broilers when subjected to chronic stress, in bioeconomic terms, and also because it favours wetter faeces.
2- Both early heat conditioning and electrolyte balance were not effective in adapting broilers to chronic stress, but rations with EE reduced the mortality of broilers subjected to heat stress.
3- Treatments with CTP resulted in paler carcasses due to the birds' longer exposure to high temperatures while alive.

CHAPTER 8

REFERENCES

AHMAD, T.; SARWAR, M. Dietary electrolyte balance: implications in heat stressed broilers. **World's Poultry Science Journal,** v. 62, n.4, p. 638-653, 2006.

ARAÚJO, W. A. G.; ROSTAGNO, H. S.; ALBINO, L. F. T.; CARVALHO T. A.; NETO A. C. R. Potassium in animal nutrition. **Revista Eletrônica Nutritime,** v.7, n. 4, p.1280-1291, 2010.

AVILA, V. S.; MAZZUCO, H.: FIGUEIREDO, E. A. P. **Poultry litter: materials, reuse, use as food and fertiliser.** EMBRAPA-CNPSA, Concórdia - SC, 1992. 38p. (EMBRAPA-CNPSA. Technical Circular, 16).

BARBOSA FILHO, J.A.D. **Evaluation of the welfare of laying hens in different production systems and environmental conditions, using image analysis.** Piracicaba - SP, 2004. Dissertation (master's degree) - University of São Paulo. 141f.. Available at: <www.teses.usp.br/teses/disponiveis/11/11131/tde-11052005-144156/publico/jose.pdf>. Accessed on 10 March 2015.

BELAY, T.; TEETER, R. G. Broiler water balance and thermobalance during thermoneutral and high ambient temperature exposure. **Poultry Science,** v.72. p.116-124. 1993.

BENTON, C.E.; BALNAVE, D.; BRAKE, J. Review: the use of dietary minerals during heat stress in broilers. **The Professional Animal Scientist,** v. 14, p. 193196, 1998.

BIANCHI, M.; PETRACCI, M.; SIRRI, F.; FOLEGATTI, E.; FRANCHINI, A.; MELUZZI, A. The influence of the season and market class of broiler chickens. **Poultry Science,** v. 86, p. 959-963, 2007.

BORGATTI, L.M.O.; ALBUQUERQUE, R.; MEISTER, N.C.; SOUZA, L.M.O.; LIMA, F.R.; TRINDADE NETO, M.A. Performance of broilers fed diets with different dietary electrolyte balance under summer conditions. **Brazilian Journal of Poultry Science**, v. 6, p. 153-157, 2004.

BORGES, S.A. Application of the electrolyte balance concept for poultry. In: APINCO CONFERENCE ON Poultry Science and Technology. **Proceedings...** Santos-SP: APINCO, 2006.p.123-137.

BORGES, S.A. **Potassium chloride and sodium bicarbonate supplementation for broilers during the summer**. Jaboticabal, 84p. Dissertation (master's degree) - Universidade Estadual Paulista Júlio.1997.

BORGES, S.A.; MAIORKA, A.; SILVA, A.V.F. Physiology of heat stress and electrolyte utilisation in broilers. **Ciência Rural**, v. 33, p. 975-981, 2003.

BORGES, S.A.; ARIKI, J.; MARTINS, C.L.; MORAES, V.M.B. Potassium chloride supplementation for broilers submitted to heat stress. **Revista Brasileira de Zootecnia**, v. 28, p. 313-319, 1999.

BRAZIL. Ministry of Agriculture, Livestock and Supply. **Poultry**. Brasília 2015. Available at <http://www.agricultura.gov.br/animal/especies/aves>. Accessed on 10 January 2015.

CASADO, E.S.; VÍRSEDA, T.A. Influencia de los minerales y otros nutrientes sobre la humedad de las deyecciones de los broilers. In: WSPA Spanish Section Symposium, 21, 1983. Barcelona. **Proceedings... Barcelona:WSPA,** 1983. p.333-338.

CHENG, T.K.; HAMRE, M.L.; COON, C.N. Responses of broilers to dietary protein levels and amino acid supplementation to low protein diets at various environmental temperatures. **Journal of Applied Poultry Research**, v.6, p.18- 33, 1997.

COBB. **Broiler handling manual.** Cobb-Ventress Brazil, 2014. 66p. Available at <http://www.cobb-vantress.com/docs/default- source/guides/broiler-managment-guide-portuguese>. Accessed on 18 February 2015.

COELLO, C.L.; MENOCAL, J.A.; GONZÁLEZ, E.A. Metabolic syndromes in broilers. In: Poultry Science and Technology. **Anais**..., Santos - SP: APINCO, 2008. p. 263-278.

COHEN, I.; HURWITZ, S.; BAR, A. Acid-base balance and sodium to chloride ratio in diets of laying hens. **Journal of Nutrition**, v. 102, p. 1-8, 1972.

FURLAN, R.L. Influence of temperature on broiler production. In: SIMPÓSIO BRASIL SUL DE AVICULTURA, n. 7, 2006. Chapecó. **Anais**..., Chapecó, SC, p.104-135.

GAMBA, J.P.; RODRIGUES, M.M.; GARCIA NETO, M.; PERRI, S.H.V.; FARIA JÚNIOR M.J. A; PINTO, M.F. The strategic application of electrolyte balance to minimise heat stress in broilers. **Brazilian Journal of Poultry Science**, v. 17, n.2, p 237-246, 2015.

GARCIA NETO, M. **Practical programme for formulating rations / broilersPPFR** . Available at:<http://www.foa.unesp.br/downloads/categoria.asp?CatCod=4&SubCatCod=138>. Accessed on 05 December 2014.

GARCIA NETO, M.; ALMEIDA, M.A.; PAES, C.R.; SANDRE, D.G.; FARIA-JUNIOR, M.J.A.; PINTO, M.F. Bioeconomic energy conversion: a new index option for evaluating bioeconomic performance. In: REUNIÃO ANUAL DA SOCIEDADE BRASILEIRA DE ZOOTECNIA, 49, 2012. **Proceedings**... Brasília - DF: Sociedade Brasileira de Zootecnia, 2012 (CD-ROM). Available at <https://sites.google.com/site/ppfrprogramforfeedformulation/papers>. Accessed on

05 October 2014.

GEZEN, S.S.; EREN, M.; DENIZ, G. The effect of different dietary electrolyte balances on eggshell quality in laying hens. **Revue Médicini Véterinaire**, v. 156, p. 491-497, 2005.

GONZALEZ-ESQUERRA, R.; LEESON, S. Physiological and metabolic responses of broilers to heat stress - implications for protein and amino acid nutrition. **World's Poultry Science Journal,** vol. 62, p. 282-295, 2006.

HARA, Y.; MAY, R.C.; KELLY, R.A.; MITCH, W.E. Acidosis, not azotemia, stimulates branched-chain, aminoacid catabolism in uremic rats. **Kidney International,** v.32, p.808-814, 1987.

HAYDON, K.D.; WEST, J.W. Effect of dietary electrolyte balance on nutrient digestibility determined at the end of the small intestine and over the total digestive tract in growing pigs. **Journal of Animal** Science, v. 68, p. 3687-3693, 1990.

JOHNSON R.J.; KARUNAJEEWA, H. The effects of dietary minerals and electrolytes on the growth and physiology of the young chick. **Journal of Nutrition,** v. 115, p. 1680-1690, 1985.

JUDICE, J.P.M.; BERTECHINI, A.G.; MUNIZ, J.A. Cation-anion balance of rations and feeding management for second cycle layers. Lavras. **Ciência Agrotécnica,** v.26, n.3, p.598-609, 2002.

JUNQUEIRA, O.M.; MILES, R.D.; HARMS, R.H. Interrelationship between phosphorus, sodium and chloride in the diet of laying hens. **Poultry Science,** v. 63, p. 1229-1236, 1984.

LEESON S.; DIAZ G.J.; SUMMERS J.D. **Metabolic disorders and mycotoxins.** Guelph:

Ontario. University Books, 1995. p. 352.

LEWIS, K.; LEITL, G.; HEINE, M. Influence of dietary potassium and sodium/potassium molar ratios on the development of salt hypertension. **The Journal of Experimental Medicine**, v. 136, p. 318-330, 1972.

LUTZ, J. Calcium balance acid-base status of women as affected by increased protein intake and by sodium bicarbonate ingestion. **The american journal of clinical nutrition**, v.39, p. 281-288, 1984.

MACARI, M. **Water in industrial poultry farming**. Jaboticabal: FUNEP, 1996. p. 128.

MACARI, M.; FURLAN, R.L.; GONZALES, E. **Avian physiology applied to broilers**. Jaboticabal: FUNEP, 1994. p. 296.

MINELLO, M.C.S.; ALMEIDA, M.A.; SANDRE, D.G.; GARCIA NETO, M.; FARIA JUNIOR, M.J.A.; PINTO, M.F. Electrolyte balance and thermal conditioning: reducing acute heat stress in broiler chickens. Botucatu - SP. **Veterinária e Zootecnia**. v.19, p. 136-137, 2012.

MINOLTA, K. **Precise colour communication. 2007.** Available at <www.konicaminolta.com/instruments/knowledge/color/pdf/color communication.pdf>. Accessed on 15 October 2014.

MONGIN, P. Recent advances in dietary anion-cation balance: application in poultry. **The Proceednigs of the Nutrition Society**, v. 40, p. 285-294, 1981.

MONGIN, P.; SAUVEUR. B. Interrelationships between mineral nutrition, acid-base balance, growth and cartilage abnormalities. In: Boorman, K.N.; Wilson,B. (ed.). **Growth and poultry meat production.** 1977, Edinburgh. Edinburgh: British Poultry

Science, 1977. p. 235-247.

MOREIRA, J. Causes of PSE meat in broilers and how to control them. In: **SEMINÁRIO INTERNACIONAL DE AVES E SUÍNOS, 4., 2005. Florianópolis. Proceedings... Florianópolis: AVESUI, 2005. p. 71-118.**

NGOKA, D. A.; FRONING, G. W. Effect of free struggle and preslaughter excitement on colour of turkey breast muscles. **Poultry Science**, v. 61, p 22912293, 1982.

NOBAKHT, A.; SHIVAZAD, M.; CHAMANY, M.; SAFAMEHER, A.R. The effects of dietary electrolyte balance on performance of laying hens exposed to heat - stress environment in late laying period. **International Journal of Poultry Science**, v. 5, n. 10, p. 955-958, 2006.

NORTHCUTT, J.K.; FOEGEDING, E.A.; EDENS, F.W. Water-holding properties of thermally preconditioned chicken breast and leg meat. **Poultry Science**, v.73, p.308-316, 1994.

NRC - National Research Council. **Nutrient requirements of poultry**. 9th ed. Washington (DC): National Academy Press, 1994. 155p.

OLIVEIRA, E.C.O.; MURAKAMI, A.E.; FRANCO, J.R.G.; CELLA, P.S.; SOUZA, L.M.G. Effect of electrolyte balance and poultry by-products on broiler performance in the initial phase (1-21 days of age). **Acta Scientiarum Animal Sciences**, v. 25, p. 293-299, 2003.

OLIVEIRA, G. C.; MOREIRA, I.; FURLAN, A. C. Effect of low crude protein diets supplemented with amino acids for castrated male piglets (15 to 30 kg). **Revista Brasileira de Zootecnia**, v. 33, n. 6, p. 17471757, 2004.

PATIENCE, J.F. A review of the role of acid-base balance in amino acid nutrition. **Journal of Animal Science**, v. 68, p. 398-408, 1990.

PATIENCE, J.F.; AUSTIC, R.E.; BOYD, R.D. Effect of dietary electrolyte balance on growth and acid-base status in swine. **Journal of Animal Science,** v. 64, p. 457-466, 1987.

PESTI, G.M. Response surface approach to studying the protein and energy requeriments of laying hens. **Poultry Science,** v.70,p103-14, 1991.

PESTI, G.M.; MILLER, B.R. Animal feed formulation: user friendly feed formulation programme. Athens: Kluwer Academic Publishers Group, 1992. p. 166.

REDDY, G.S.; JONES, G.; KOOH, S.W.; FRASER, D. Inhibition of 25-hydroxyvitamin D3-1-hydroxylase by chronic metabolic acidosis. **American Journal of Physiology**, v. 243, p. 265-E271, 1982.

RIDDEL, C. Studies on the pathogenesis of tibial dyschondroplasia in chickens. II. Growth rate of long bones. **Avian Diseases,** v.19, p.490-496, 1975.

RODRIGUES, M.I.; IEMMA, A.F. **Planning experiments and optimising processes.** 2 ed. 358 p.

ROSS, J.G.; SPEARS, J.W.; GARLICH, J.D. Dietary electrolyte balance effects on performance and metabolic characteristics in finishing steers. **Jounal of Animal Science,** v. 72, p. 1600-1607, 1994.

ROSTAGNO, H.S.; ALBINO,L.F.T.; DONZELE, J.L.; GOMES, P.C.; OLIVEIRA, R.F.; LOPES, D.C.; FERREIRA, A.S.; BARRETO, S.L.T.; EUCLIDES, R.F. **Brazilian tables for poultry and pigs:** food composition and nutritional requirements. 3.ed. Viçosa: UFV, Department of Animal Science, 2011. 252p. Available at <http://cienciaavicola.com.br/teste/public_html/pdf/02-TABELAS- BRASILEIRAS-AVES-E-SUINOS-2011 .pdf.>. Accessed on 12 February 2015.

RUTZ, F. Physiological aspects that regulate thermal comfort in poultry. In:

CONFERÊNCIA APINCO DE CIÊNCIA E TECNOLOGIA AVÍCOLA, **Anais**... Santos - SP: APINCO, 1994. p.73-84.

SAS Institute. **SAS® users guide**: statistics. 5. ed. Cary: SAS Institute, Inc., 2009.

SAVEUR, B. Dietary factors as causes of leg abnomalities in poultry - a review. **World's Poultry Science Journal**, v.40, p. 195-206, 1984.

SAVEUR, B.; MONGIN, P. Interrationships between dietary concentrations of sodium, potassium and chloride in laying hens. **Brazilian Poultry Science**, v.19, p. 475-485, 1978.

SILVA, D. J.; QUEIROZ, A. C. **Food analysis - chemical and biological methods**. 3. ed. Viçosa: Ed. UFV, 2002. p. 235.

SMITH, M.O.; TEETER, R.G. Potassium balance of the5 to 8-week-old broiler exposed to constant heat or cycling high temperature stress and the effects of supplemental potassium chloride on body weight gain and feed efficiency. **Poultry Science**, v. 66, p. 487-492. 1987.

SMITH, M.O.; TEETER, R.G. Effect of ammonium chloride and potassium chloride on survival of broiler chicks during acute heat stress. **Nutrition Research**, v.7, p.677-681, 1987

SOUZA, B.B.; BERTECHINI, A.G.; TEIXEIRA, A.S.; LIMA, J.A.F.; FREITAS, R.T.F. Effect of potassium chloride supplementation in the diet on the acid-base balance and performance of broilers in summer. **Ciência Agrotecnologia**, v. 26, p. 1297-1304, 2002.

TALBOT, C.J. Sodium, potassium and chloride imbalance in broiler diets. **The Proceedinigs of Nutrition Society**, v. 37, p. 53A, 1978.

TAKAHASHI, S.E. **Occurrence of pale meat and quality characteristics of broiler meat.** Botucatu - SP, 2007, Unesp, 86f. Thesis (PhD in Zootechnics) - Department of Animal Production, Faculty of Veterinary Medicine and Zootechnics. Available at <http://livros01.livrosgratis.com.br/cp033239.pdf.>. Accessed on 13 April 2015.

TEETER, R.G.; SMITH, M.O.; OWENS, F.N.; ARP, S.C.; SANGIAH, S.; BREAZILE, J.E. Chronic heat stress and respiratory alkalosis: occurrence and treatment in broiler chicks. **Poultry Science**, v. 64, p. 1060-1064, 1985.

THORP, B.H.; DUCRO, B.; WHITEHEAD, C.C. Avian tibial dyschondroplasia: the interaction of genetic selection and dietary 1,25-dihydroxycholecalciferol. **Avian Pathology**, v.22, p.311-324, 1993.

VIEIRA, B.S. **Influence of early thermal conditioning and daily photoperiod on the performance and thermal tolerance of broilers in the final phase of rearing.** 2008. 53 f. Dissertation (Master's Degree) - Universidade Estadual Paulista "Júlio de Mesquita Filho" Faculdade de Ciências Agrárias e Veterinárias. Jaboticabal, São Paulo.

VIEITES, F. M.; MORAES, G.H.K.; ALBINO, L.F.T.; ROSTAGNO, H.S.; ATENCIO, A.; VARGAS JUNIOR, J.G. Electrolyte balance and crude protein levels on performance, carcass yield and litter moisture of broilers from 1 to 42 days of age. **Revista Brasileira de Zootecnia,** v.34, n.6, p.1990-1999, 2005.

VIEITES, F.M.; MORAES, G.H.K.; ALBINO, L.F.T.; ROSTAGNO, H.S.; RODRIGUES, A.C.; SILVA, F.A.; ATENCIO, A. Electrolyte balance and crude protein levels on blood and bone parameters of broilers at 21 days of age. **Revista Brasileira de Zootecnia,** v.33, p.1520-1530, 2004.

YAHAV, S.; HURWITZ, S. Induction of thermotolerance in male broiler chickens by temperature conditioning at an early age. **Poultry Science,** v.75, p.402-406, 1996.

YAHAV, S.; McMURTRY, J. P. Thermotolerance acquisition in broiler chickens by temperature conditioning early in life - the effect of timing and ambient temperature. **Poultry Science,** v.80, p. 1662-1666, 2001.

WILDMAN, C. D.; WEST, J. W.; BERNARD, J. K. Effects of dietary cation-anion difference and potassium to sodium ratio on lactating dairy cows in hot weather. **Journal of Dairy Science,** v. 90, p. 970-977, 2007.

WOELFEL, R. L.; OWENS, C. M. ; HIRSCHLER, E. M.; MARTINEZ-DAWSON, R.; SAMS, A. R. The Characterisation and Incidence of Pale, Soft, and Exudative Broiler Meat in a Commercial Processing Plant. **Poultry Science,** v. 81, p.579- 584, 2002.

CHAPTER 9

APPENDIX

A - PHOTOS OF THE EXPERIMENT

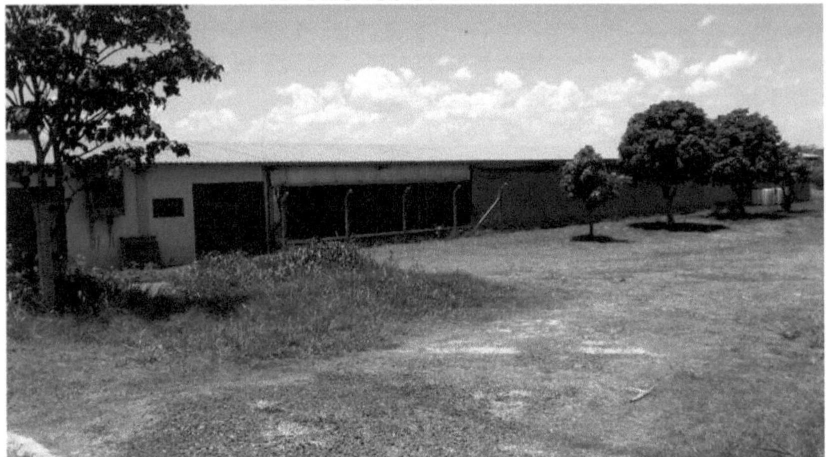

Figure 1A - Experimental Zootechnics Sector of the Faculty of Medicine Veterinary - UNESP - Araçatuba.

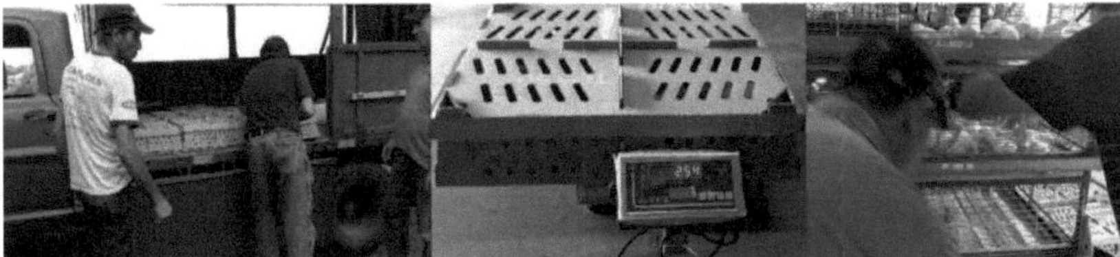

Figure 2A - Arrival, weighing and random distribution of the chicks.

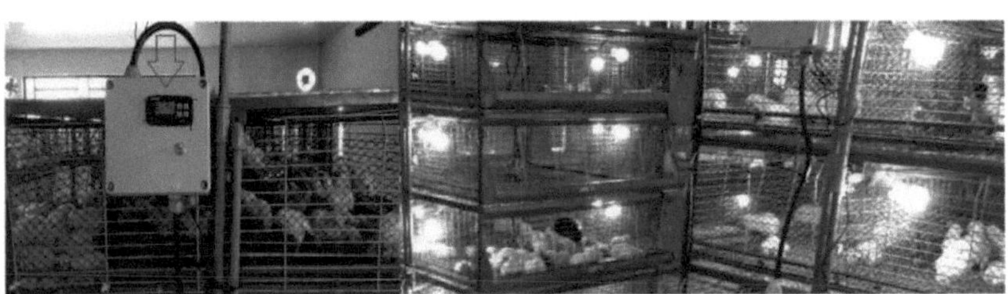

Figure 3A - Birds in batteries during TCP application (24 h at 36 C)

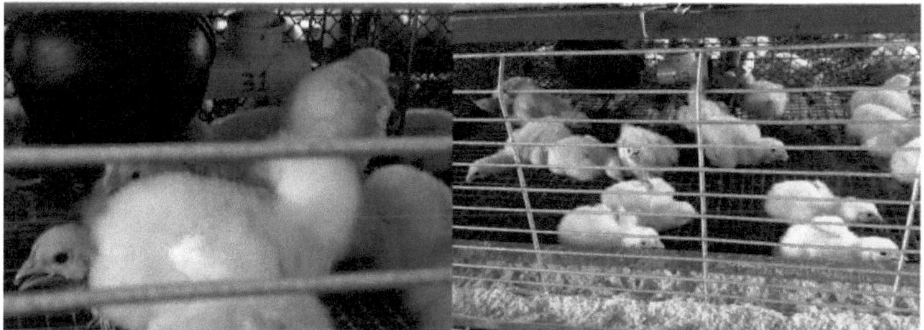

Figure 4A - Birds gasping for breath during TCP application.

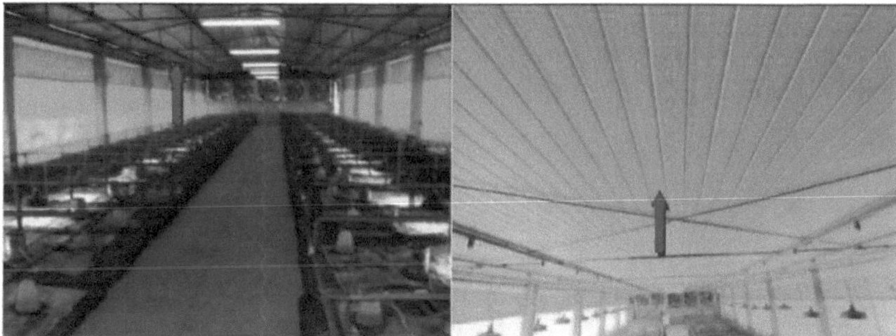

Figure 5A - Before and after lining the shed for better environmental control.

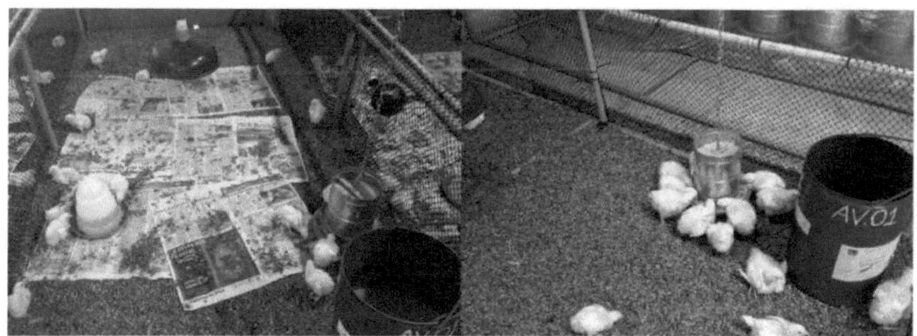

Figure 6A - An experimental plot with 20 birds in a box.

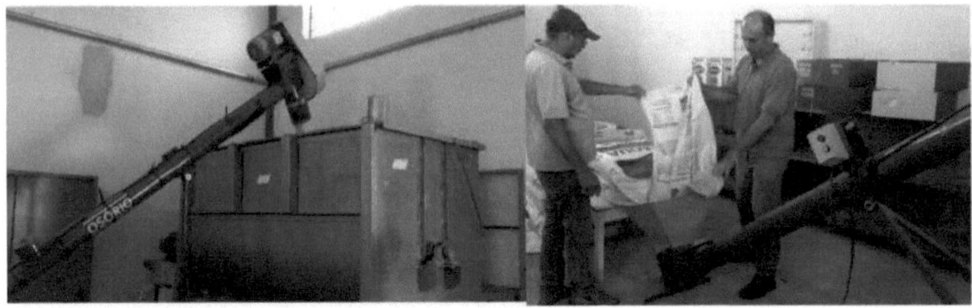

Figure 7A - Feed churning at the Zootechnics Experimental Sector Factory of the University of Coimbra

Faculty of Veterinary Medicine - UNESP - Araçatuba.

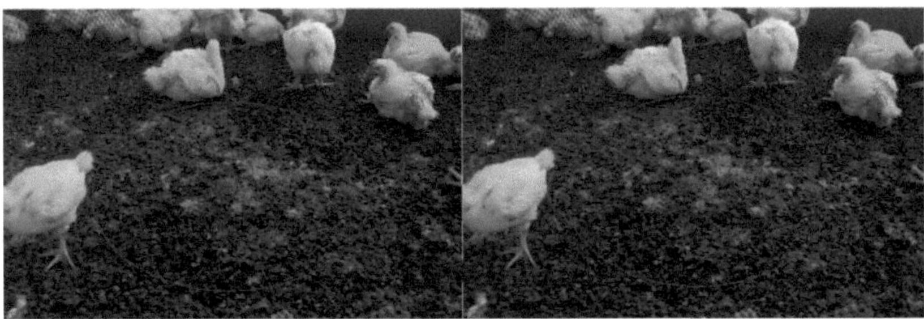

Figure 8A - Damp litter due to high humidity from bird faeces.

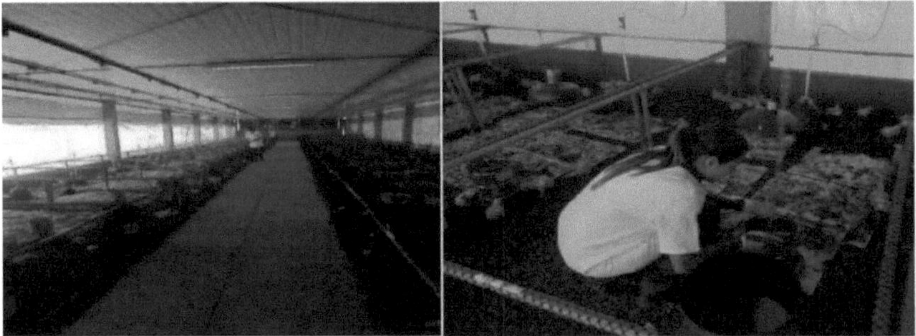

Figure 9A - Experimental shed and master's student replacing feed in the feeders.

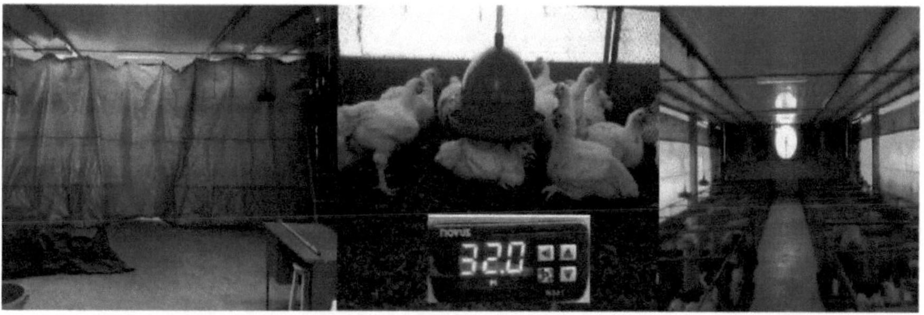

Figure 10A - Application of chronic heat stress from the 35th to the 39th day of life (5 days/ 6 hours a day/ 32°C).

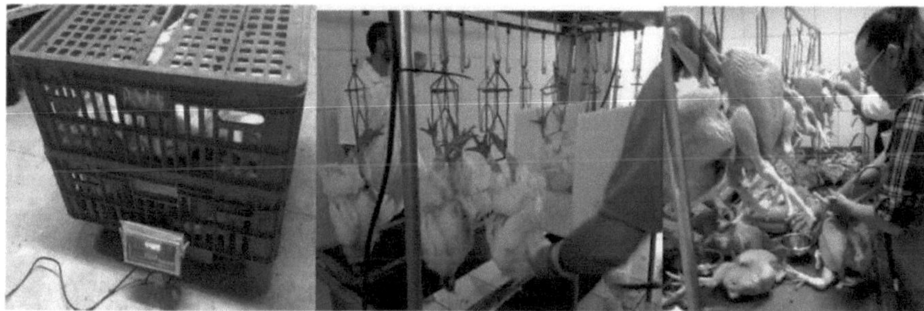

Figure 11A - Weighing and slaughter of the birds on the 42nd day of life.

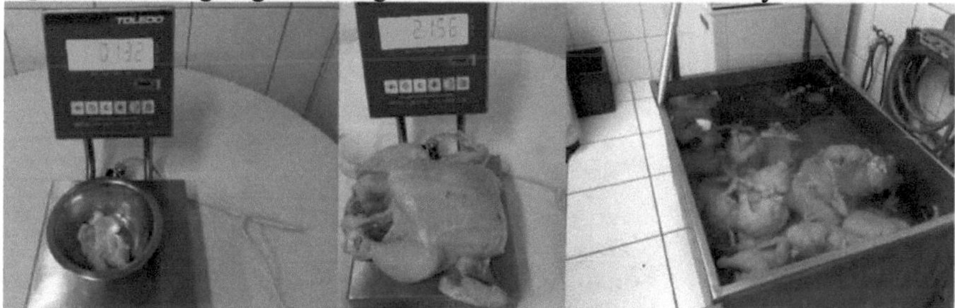

Figure 12A - Abdominal fat weighing, clean carcass weighing and carcasses in the chiller.

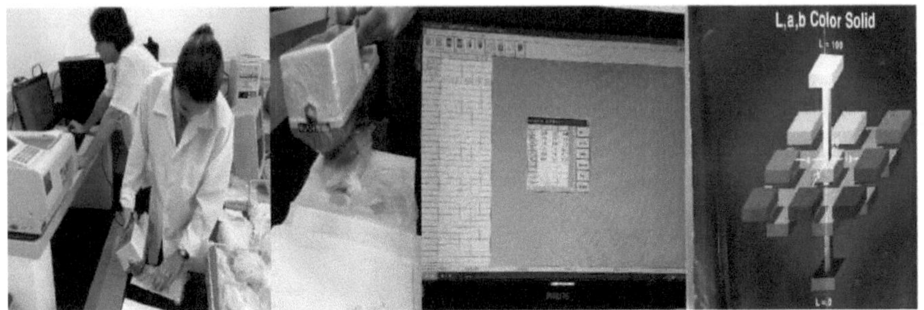

Figure 13A - Master's student performing breast colour analysis with MiniScan XE Plus

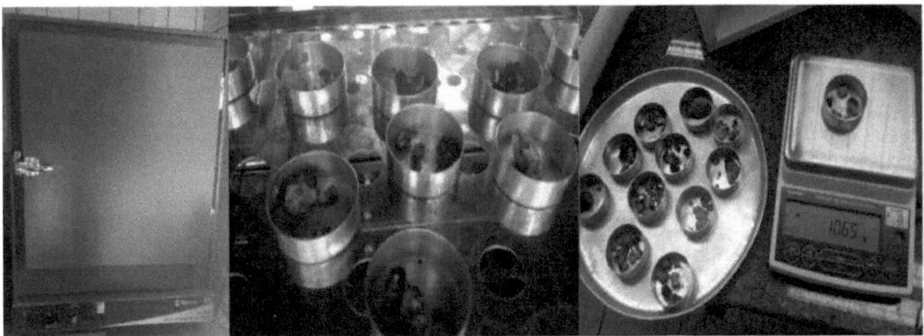

Figure 14A - Faeces analysis.

ANNEX B - SPREADSHEET FOR CALCULATING FEED CONSUMPTION AND FEED CONVERSION CORRECTED FOR MORTALITY

Data	07/abr	08/abr	09/abr	10/abr	11/abr	12/abr	13/abr	14/abr	15/abr	16/abr	17/abr	18/abr	19/abr	20/abr	21/abr	22/abr	23/abr	24/abr	25/abr	26/abr	27/abr	28/abr	A Total de ave	B Consumo de ração	B/A = C Consumo ave/dia	C*21 = D Consumo corrigido	E Peso médio ave	D/E Conversão corrigida
BOX	0	1	2	3	4	5	6	7	8	9	10	11	12	13	14	15	16	17	18	19	20	21						
1	20	20	20	20	20	20	19	19	19	19	19	19	19	19	19	19	19	19	19	19	19	19	404	23	0,06	1,20	0,93	1,28
2	20	20	19	19	19	18	17	17	17	17	17	17	17	17	17	17	17	17	17	17	17	17	367	21,98	0,07	1,43	0,95	1,51
3	20	20	20	20	19	19	19	19	18	18	18	18	18	18	18	18	18	18	18	18	18	18	386	23,78	0,06	1,29	0,97	1,33
4	20	20	20	20	20	20	20	20	20	20	20	20	20	20	20	20	20	20	20	20	20	20	420	23,89	0,06	1,19	0,84	1,43
5	20	20	20	20	19	19	18	18	18	18	18	18	18	18	18	18	18	18	18	18	18	18	386	22,88	0,06	1,24	1,00	1,24
6	20	20	20	20	20	19	19	19	19	19	19	19	19	19	19	19	19	19	19	19	19	19	403	23,32	0,06	1,22	0,91	1,34
7	20	20	20	20	20	20	19	19	19	19	19	19	19	19	19	19	19	19	19	19	19	18	403	22,81	0,06	1,19	0,92	1,29
8	20	20	20	20	20	20	20	20	20	20	20	20	20	20	20	20	20	19	19	19	19	19	416	23,48	0,06	1,19	0,91	1,30
9	20	20	20	18	18	18	18	18	18	17	17	17	17	17	17	17	17	17	17	17	17	16	368	20,16	0,05	1,15	0,90	1,28
10	20	20	20	20	20	20	20	20	20	20	20	20	20	20	20	20	20	20	20	20	20	19	419	24,64	0,06	1,23	0,86	1,43
11	20	20	20	19	19	19	19	19	19	19	19	19	19	19	19	19	19	19	19	19	19	18	400	23,88	0,06	1,25	0,91	1,37
12	20	20	20	20	20	19	19	19	19	19	19	19	19	19	19	19	19	19	19	19	19	19	403	24,49	0,06	1,28	0,93	1,37
13	20	20	20	20	19	19	19	19	19	19	19	19	19	19	19	19	19	19	19	19	19	19	402	24,07	0,06	1,26	0,88	1,42
14	20	20	20	20	20	20	20	20	20	20	19	20	20	20	20	20	20	20	20	20	20	20	419	24,18	0,06	1,21	0,95	1,27
15	20	20	19	19	18	18	17	17	17	17	17	16	16	16	16	16	16	16	16	16	16	16	356	18,35	0,05	1,09	0,84	1,30
16	20	20	19	19	19	19	19	19	19	18	18	17	17	17	17	17	17	17	17	17	17	17	376	21,56	0,06	1,20	0,91	1,33
17	20	20	20	20	20	20	20	20	20	20	20	20	20	20	20	20	19	19	19	19	19	19	414	24,27	0,06	1,23	0,93	1,33
18	20	20	20	19	19	19	18	18	18	18	18	17	17	17	17	17	17	17	17	17	17	16	373	21,29	0,06	1,20	0,80	1,49
19	20	20	20	20	20	20	20	20	20	20	20	20	20	20	20	20	20	20	20	20	20	20	420	24,75	0,06	1,24	0,85	1,45
20	20	20	19	19	19	19	19	19	19	18	18	17	17	17	17	17	17	17	17	17	17	17	376	22,96	0,06	1,28	0,94	1,36
21	20	20	20	19	19	19	19	19	19	19	19	19	19	19	19	19	19	19	19	19	19	18	400	24,43	0,06	1,28	1,03	1,25
22	20	20	19	19	18	18	18	17	17	17	17	17	17	17	17	17	17	17	17	17	17	17	367	22,53	0,06	1,29	0,92	1,41
23	20	20	20	20	20	20	20	20	20	20	20	20	20	20	20	20	20	20	20	20	20	20	420	25,05	0,06	1,25	0,92	1,37
24	20	20	20	19	19	19	18	17	17	17	17	17	17	17	17	17	17	17	17	17	17	17	370	20,29	0,05	1,15	0,85	1,39
25	20	20	20	20	20	20	20	19	19	19	19	19	19	19	19	19	18	18	18	18	18	18	399	23,6	0,06	1,24	0,92	1,35
26	20	20	20	20	20	20	20	20	20	20	20	20	20	20	20	20	20	20	20	20	20	20	420	24,46	0,06	1,22	0,88	1,39
27	20	20	20	20	20	20	20	20	20	20	20	20	20	20	20	20	20	20	20	20	20	20	420	24,76	0,06	1,24	0,93	1,33
28	20	20	20	20	20	20	20	20	20	20	20	20	20	20	20	20	20	20	20	20	20	20	420	23,98	0,06	1,20	0,89	1,35
29	20	20	20	19	18	18	18	18	18	18	18	18	18	17	17	17	17	17	17	17	17	17	374	19,79	0,05	1,11	0,86	1,29
30	20	20	19	19	18	18	18	17	17	17	17	17	17	17	17	17	17	17	17	17	17	17	367	21,11	0,06	1,21	0,89	1,36
31	20	20	20	20	20	20	20	20	20	20	20	20	20	20	20	20	20	20	20	20	20	20	420	24,33	0,06	1,22	1,17	1,04
32	20	20	20	20	20	20	19	18	18	18	18	18	18	18	18	18	18	18	18	18	18	18	389	22,2	0,06	1,20	0,91	1,31

Figure 1B - Mortality annotation table for adjusting consumption and feed conversion in the initial phase (at 21 days).

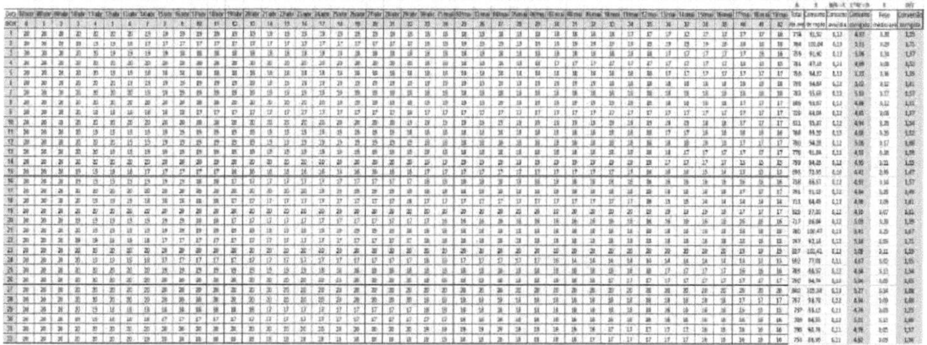

Figure 2 B - Mortality annotation table for adjusting consumption and feed conversion in the finishing phase (at 42 days).

ANNEX C - BIOECONOMIC ENERGY CONVERSION INDEX (BEC) SPREADSHEET

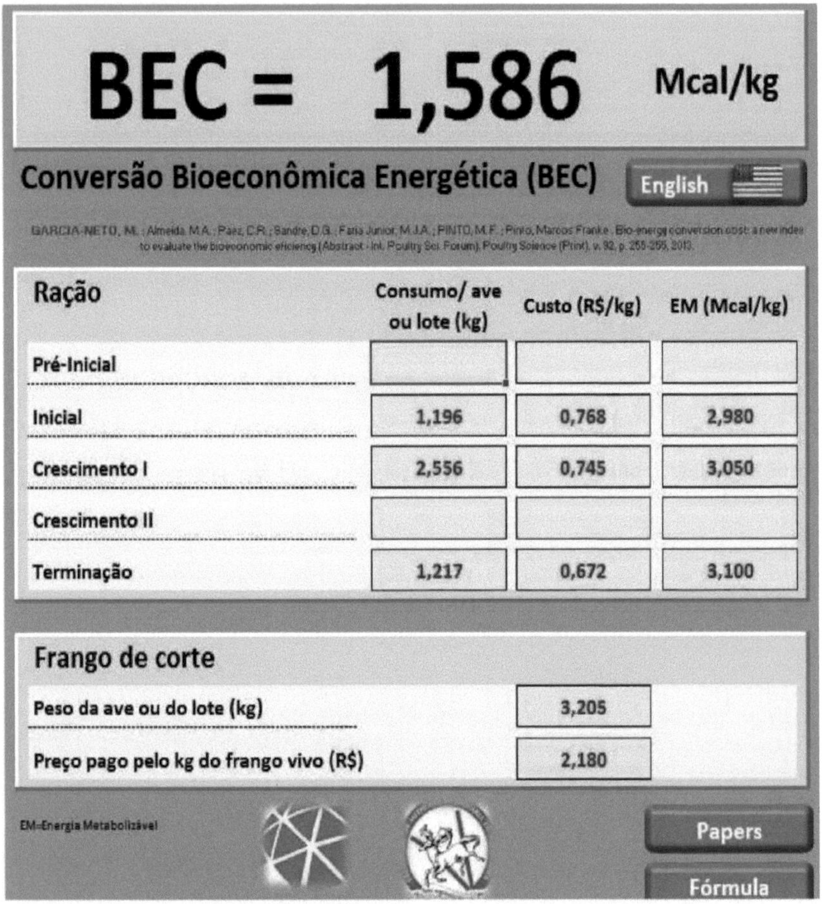

BEC = 1,586 Mcal/kg

Conversão Bioeconômica Energética (BEC)

English

GARCIA-NETO, M.; Almeida M.A.; Paez, C.R.; Sandre, D.G.; Faria Junior, M.J.A.; PINTO, M.F.; Pinto, Marcos Franke. Bio-energy conversion cost: a new index to evaluate the bioeconomic efficiency (Abstract - Int. Poultry Sci. Forum). Poultry Science (Print), v. 92, p. 255-255, 2013.

Ração	Consumo/ ave ou lote (kg)	Custo (R$/kg)	EM (Mcal/kg)
Pré-Inicial			
Inicial	1,196	0,768	2,980
Crescimento I	2,556	0,745	3,050
Crescimento II			
Terminação	1,217	0,672	3,100

Frango de corte	
Peso da ave ou do lote (kg)	3,205
Preço pago pelo kg do frango vivo (R$)	2,180

EM=Energia Metabolizável

Papers

Fórmula

Figure 1C - BEC spreadsheet available at:
https://sites.google.com/site/ppfrparaexcel2007ousuperior/papers

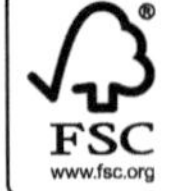

MIX
Papier aus verantwortungsvollen Quellen
Paper from responsible sources
FSC® C105338

Printed by Books on Demand GmbH, Norderstedt / Germany